The Adrenal Reset Power Boost Diet

How to Stop Feeling Tired, Stressed, Fatigued & Irritable and Learn to Balance Your Hormones!

Jamie Sandulf

DEDICATION

This book is dedicated to everyone who has ever known that she was suffering from an illness but had difficulty getting her doctors to diagnose it. I especially want to dedicate this book to all of those who have struggled from adrenal fatigue and are ready to take back their lives from this energy-draining sickness.

CONTENTS

1 INTRODUCTION

If you have purchased this book I have to assume that you may be feeling run down and tired, but cannot attribute it to any specific reason. Even though you might be getting enough sleep, you still have difficulties waking up and getting out of bed in the mornings. Do you keep hitting the snooze button on the alarm to go back to sleep for "just ten more minutes?"

During the day you may be drinking several cups of coffee, or drinking a few cans of soft drinks, or even consuming several Red Bull® or similar energy drinks to try to stay alert throughout the day.

Do you find yourself craving salty or sweet

snacks?

Do your family members and close friends ever tell you that you seem to be in a bad mood or are cranky?

If the above situations sound familiar, then it is possible you are one of the estimated 80% of the North American population who have experienced adrenal fatigue or the symptoms of stress at one time or another in their lives.

In this e-book, not only will you find an explanation as to how and why the adrenal gland may be responsible for creating symptoms of stress, but you will also learn proven steps and strategies for taking back your life, feeling better, resetting your hormones and regaining your energy!

I want to thank you for purchasing this book, "The Adrenal Reset Power Boost: How to Stop Feeling Tired, Stressed, Fatigued & Irritable and Learn to Balance Your Hormones!" It is the first step on your path of recovery.

2 WHAT ARE THE TRUE REASONS YOU HAVE THESE SYMPTOMS?

Sometimes annoying and unexplainable symptoms haunt us. We may feel weird body aches, unable to concentrate, moodiness or irritability, feel very tired, experience racing thoughts or unexpected cravings for sweet or salty foods. These symptoms may not be bad enough to send us to the doctor, or we may even dismiss them as the effects of aging or just being tired – but when they start to affect our everyday activities and become chronic symptoms, then there may be cause for alarm.

According to Dr. James Wilson, author of the book "Adrenal Fatigue: The 21st Century Stress Syndrome," people may not know that malfunctioning adrenal glands can be the culprit for these unexpected symptoms (along with others that are related to adrenal fatigue). Dr. Wilson has stated that for most people, adrenal fatigue can be relieved with the proper care. If you are suffering from any of the aforementioned symptoms, you can expect to feel better if you get support for your condition, promote healthy adrenal function and, most of all, reduce your stress.

The truth about adrenal fatigue

If you research adrenal fatigue, you will notice that most of the information you find is either unsupported or contradicts the theory that adrenal fatigue may be the reason behind a variety of health conditions.

People who have sought their doctor's advice for adrenal fatigue have been told that it is not an acknowledged medical condition. There are no drugs to cure adrenal fatigue and, therefore, it is not considered to be part of a conventional medical model. But what people fail to understand is that these nagging symptoms are the body's way of signaling that there is an imbalance. Some ignore the signs or dismiss them and go on with their everyday life. However, for some the symptoms may be very hard to totally overlook.

Prolonged sleeplessness can lead to insomnia and may affect your work, career and your personal relationships. Feeling fatigued and having poor concentration can lead to poor judgment and lack of energy at work and in school. When you ignore adrenal fatigue symptoms, everything important in your life eventually becomes affected.

You need a power boost!

If you are tired of being tired, weak from feeling weak for a long time, then this is the best time to start reviving your life. You can regain your energy and enjoy many of the following benefits when you adopt a Reset Power Boost Diet that is especially designed for people suffering from adrenal fatigue:

- Say goodbye to annoying body aches and start moving again

- Improve your concentration and have a sharper memory

- Improve your mood allowing you to enjoy your life better

- Improve your energy levels

- Correct hormonal imbalances

- Reduce cravings and improve your appetite

The Adrenal Reset Power Boost Diet is a totally new dietary approach to correcting adrenal fatigue. This book will guide you on how this kind of diet can help you regain normal adrenal function and will provide you with amazing energy to power up your day.

There is hope for adrenal fatigue! Let's start making a change now!

3 WHAT ARE THE ADRENAL GLANDS?

To fully understand what adrenal fatigue is and how an Adrenal Reset Power Boost Diet works, you must first learn about the adrenal glands.

Little is actually known about the adrenal glands, they come up in healthcare literature less frequently than other endocrine glands such as the thyroid glands and pituitary glands. Even so, the adrenal glands perform several vital functions that are important for the body's normal metabolic functions. The adrenal glands look like two triangular-shaped organs. Each of these measures around 1.5 inches x 3 inches.

HUMAN KIDNEYS

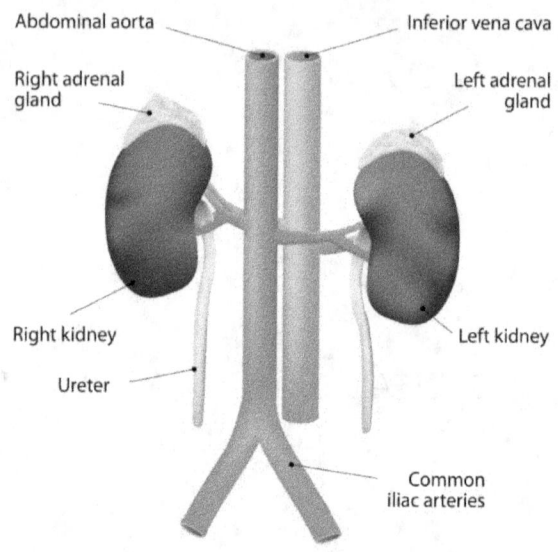

Identifying the Adrenal glands

The functions of the adrenal glands

The adrenal glands are located on top of your kidneys. Each kidney has an adrenal gland with two basic parts. Each part has a special function:

1. The adrenal cortex is the outer part of the adrenal glands. It is responsible for producing cortisol (a hormone that

> regulates metabolism and stress response) and aldosterone (a hormone that helps control blood pressure).

2. The adrenal medulla is the inner part and this produces adrenaline which is important in the body's reaction to stress.

Adrenal glands may produce more or less hormones than you actually need. Having more or less hormones can make you feel uneasy, or even sick. Often, this kind of condition happens during pregnancy, or is a congenital condition. However there are also malfunctions of the adrenal gland that can develop later in life.

Diseases associated with the adrenal glands

The adrenal glands can fail due to infections, tumors and disorders of the immune system. The body may have more or less amounts of hormones than the gland normally secretes and this can lead to a variety of medical conditions. Treatment for these conditions varies according to the severity of symptoms; oftentimes the patient is prescribed medication or may even be advised to undergo surgery.

Adrenal fatigue, on the other hand, is a condition brought about by burnout of the glands. It happens when the adrenal glands can't keep up with the stress that the body is experiencing.

Controlling adrenal fatigue is different from treating adrenal failure. The main focus is to reduce stress, eat a diet designed to keep the adrenal glands healthy, and, in some cases, take adrenal fatigue supplements. Proponents of wellness also believe that exposure to pollution and toxins can also lead to overworked adrenal glands. Therefore eating natural foods that are free from chemicals and contaminants is one of the best ways to promote adrenal health.

4 A CLOSER LOOK AT ADRENAL FATIGUE

Adrenal fatigue can happen to anyone but adults are the most prone. You may have the condition but have dismissed it as just feeling tired, stressed or overworked. Some people may even overlook adrenal fatigue symptoms as signs of menopause or simply getting old.

Definition

Adrenal fatigue is a collection of symptoms that occur when the adrenal glands are unable to secrete hormones as efficiently as they should. Adrenal function falls below the levels necessary to sustain the body which results in a host of symptoms.

Adrenal fatigue has been known by many names since it was first discovered. The most common are non-Addison's hypoadrenia, neurasthenia, adrenal neurasthenia, adrenal apathy and sub-clinical hypoadrenia. This condition affects millions of people around the world, even if conventional medicine does not consider adrenal fatigue a distinct syndrome.

Theories

Adrenal fatigue happens when the adrenal glands are unable to meet the demands of stress. These glands are responsible for regulating the body's response to stress – whether it is physical, emotional and psychological stress – through the hormones that it secretes.

Adrenal hormones are responsible for regulating the body's energy, immune function, muscle strength and tone, heart rate and the body's different processes that are used to deal with stress.

Stress varies in intensity. In one way, stress is beneficial to the body. Low-level stress can stimulate the production of neurotrophins that improve the connections between the millions of neurons in the brain. Therefore it can boost brainpower. Stress can also make you more resilient or even motivate you to succeed in various activities.

However, high-level stress can negatively affect

the body. Major emotional stresses, such as a death in the family or a change in career, or physical stresses, such as a major illness or surgery, can seriously affect the body. Continual exposure to stressful situations can lead to a failure of the body to cope and adrenal fatigue.

In these circumstances, the adrenal glands do not function well enough to provide balance and this can lead to various symptoms. The output of regulatory hormones may diminish, due to over-stimulation of the glands. This may be due to a single intense stress or repeated stresses that lead to a cumulative effect.

Symptoms

There are various symptoms that tell you that you may be suffering from adrenal fatigue. Here are the most common signs and symptoms that can happen, often without any tangible reason at all:

1. You feel unusually tired.

2. You feel very tired and unable to get out of bed in the mornings. This is so even if you slept early in the evening.

3. You feel very overwhelmed and rundown.

4. You feel the urge to eat salty or sweet snacks.

5. You find it hard to bounce back from an illness or stress.

How to diagnose

There are no specific tests to diagnose adrenal fatigue. Since most of the symptoms could indicate other kinds of illnesses, it is a must for anyone who suspects that he is suffering from adrenal fatigue to monitor his symptoms.

1. Create a diary of your symptoms. Note the severity, intensity, and, if you took any kind of medication or treatment for your condition, you should note this as well.

2. Determine how often the symptoms happen.

3. Consult your doctor if you have been diagnosed with other conditions or illnesses, and if you are taking any kind of medication for your condition.

Treatments

There are several natural or wellness approaches to the treatment of adrenal fatigue. Most of these remedies are based on the premise that the condition may be brought about by chronic stress.

Reducing existing stress and preventing more stress is therefore vital for dealing with adrenal fatigue.

Stress relief

Although a small amount of stress can actually help the body become resilient and improve brain function, medium to high levels of stress may be very dangerous to the body. Whether it is acute stress or chronic stress, this negative energy wreaks havoc in the body, affecting the immune system. It can also lead to terrible psychological conditions. Not being able to cope with stress may lead to mental breakdowns, depression, or even suicide.

The five following categories of natural stress relief activities can reduce stress levels, and even prevent harmful stress in the future by helping the body adapt:

1. Relaxation activities

It's hard to even think of relaxation when your mind is racing with negative emotions. However, retreating from a stressful situation and engaging in some relaxation activities can severely reduce your discomfort. Some of the most common relaxation activities are the following:

- Drinking relaxing teas

- Aromatherapy

- Deep breathing

- Sleeping

- Spa treatments

- Getting a massage

- Walking your dog

- Playing with your children in a playground

Engaging in at least one relaxing activity each day will eventually help you to cope positively with stress. You may use any stress reduction activity as long as it does not interfere with your regular activities or schedule.

2. Yoga and meditation

Yoga and meditation help the body reduce stress by keeping the body fit and the mind healthy. Meditation is used in yoga; while performing the different poses and movements, the person is asked to concentrate and put his thoughts into the activity. Meditation also calls for engaging in yoga positions that can help improve the flow of energy in the body.

Yoga and meditation, when practiced regularly, can help reduce stress and improve mood. They can even help improve sleep and appetite. Training in yoga and meditation should be done under the guidance of an experienced instructor.

3. Physical activities and sports

Stress relief may be achieved by engaging in various physical activities and sports. A major reason for this is that the exercising body releases chemicals called endorphins that can help reduce stress and pain. There are a lot of different physical activities available to you – sports, hiking, jogging, going to the gym, aerobics exercises and dancing.

4. Turning to the outdoors

There is a great delight and sense of freedom just being in the outdoors. Simply taking pets outdoors can reduce stress and improve energy levels for both pet and owner alike. It does not matter where you go – walk on the beach, go to the park or even walk to the local mall. Get out and do anything outdoors. It's a free and easy way to reduce stress.

5. Socialization

Talking to someone in person or using social media to communicate with a friend or a family member can help reduce stress and anxiety. Humans are social creatures and we find great pleasure in talking, conversing and socializing.

Sometimes stress causes us to shut ourselves away from other people and refuse their help. Severe and chronic stress can suppress socialization skills.

The key to winning out over adrenal fatigue is to combine using relaxation and engaging in activities that divert attention with the use of a specialized diet.

The Role of Diet

Food can do a lot for increased good health and dietary strategies for wellness have been used for years. There is definitely a strong relationship between the foods we eat and the different medical conditions that we have.

For example, consider a person with diabetes. Taking drugs to manage sugar levels alone will not be enough. Creating a diet plan that will help manage sugar and nutrient intake must also be undertaken in order to successfully control the symptoms of diabetes. Along with medications and diet, exercise and a lifestyle overhaul is also required. Only when these are considered together can diabetes symptoms be fully controlled and a diabetic able to live a far healthier and better life.

Similarly, in the control of adrenal fatigue

symptoms, diet plays a huge part. Food can deliver the necessary nutrients, such as vitamins and minerals, that can improve adrenal health. Natural foods (meaning foods that does not contain chemicals, preservatives or other artificial substances designed to enhance appearance and taste) reduce toxin accumulations in the body that lead to stress. Most of all, eating the right food at the right time can greatly improves adrenal health.

The value of eating the right kind of food and using the nutrients in these foods correctly is very important for wellness. Food and diet are so important that the entire next chapter has been dedicated to the subject.

Jamie Sandulf

5 THE ADRENAL RESET POWER BOOST DIET

As mentioned earlier, diet is very important for adrenal recovery. Many foods can be used to support adrenal health. These foods do not just fill you and satiate your hunger, but will also replenish the energy you need to fuel your activity throughout the day. And there are so many more ways food can help you when dealing with health and wellness. But first, you must find out what the Adrenal Reset Power Boost Diet is all about and what this diet can do for you.

Definition

The Adrenal Reset Power Boost Diet is a new kind of diet plan created by wellness experts in the belief that adrenal fatigue may contribute to weakness, easy fatigability, depression, insomnia, inability to focus, and many other symptoms. It's a diet plan based on eating foods that support adrenal health and replenish adrenal energy. Here are a few important pointers about the Adrenal Reset Power Boost Diet:

Removing foods that are taxing your adrenal glands

Chronic and untreated stress can lead to fatigue of the adrenal glands. Therefore it makes sense to reduce any more stress to the glands. There are a lot of ways in which adrenal glands can get further stressed by eating unhealthy foods. Foods that contain preservatives, artificial flavors or colors, and chemicals should be completely avoided. Also, any fruit, vegetables, grains, or dairy products grown using fertilizers, pesticides, or fungicides should be completely avoided. Instead, look for food with a certified "Organic" label.

Adrenal glands may also become more stressed when foods that cause allergic reaction are eaten. An allergic reaction to food can overwork the immune system, and thus, tax the adrenal glands even more. A person suffering from an allergic reaction may develop hives, swelling, difficulty breathing or anxiety. All of these could make the adrenals more overworked and could worsen symptoms.

Eating fresh, natural, whole foods

Avoid preservatives, artificial flavors, dyes and chemicals used to process foods and instead, consume natural and whole foods. By doing so, you allow the adrenals space to heal.

Fresh and natural foods are safer since these are fresh from the harvest. Natural foods are free from dangerous toxins that can lead to chronic illnesses and therefore add more pressure on the adrenal glands.

Choosing food that are unprocessed

Unprocessed foods are natural foods that retain most of their nutrients and therefore help fight adrenal fatigue. Natural nutrient-dense food contains healthy amounts of fat and natural fiber and is usually low in sugar too. All of these properties help reduce pressure on the adrenal glands and improve overall health.

Processed foods include foods that are labeled as "microwavable." These foods are not only loaded with preservatives, but can be hard to digest since they contain fillers. Prepared foods with fillers wear down the body's energy stores since they are very hard for the body to break down, disrupting the cycle of digestion.

Avoiding foods with hydrogenated oils

Hydrogenated oils are highly inflammatory and can lead to inflammation of the adrenal glands. Vegetable oils such as canola, corn and soybean are the hydrogenated oils most commonly used in cooking dishes and baking. Instead, substitute healthier, "good fat" alternatives such as olive oil, coconut oil and organic butter.

Timing your meals

Spacing your meals several hours apart is one way to help the body digest the food that you eat and to fully benefit from these foods. Spacing allows the body to completely digest food and thus more efficiently absorb nutrients and digest fiber. It also reduces pressure on the adrenal glands to produce the hormones needed for the metabolism of carbohydrates, protein and fat. Should the adrenal glands be already fatigued, spacing meals ensures that the gland is not overworked.

The same goes for those occasions when we do not eat anything for a long period of time. The adrenal glands work hard to maintain the body's normal functions and release more cortisol and adrenaline during fasting. As the body's blood sugar falls during a long period of hunger, the body becomes stressed and this again affects the adrenal glands. Therefore, it is important to remember that:

1.   The body always needs energy to maintain proper function, even when it is asleep. Cortisol keeps blood sugar levels stable in between meals and at night. Therefore regulating our meals to ensure that we have reserved energy before we sleep is important.

2.   Timely and healthy small meals taken at frequent intervals throughout the day will ensure energy is distributed all day long.

3.   Timing our meals will regulate cortisol levels all throughout the day. Cortisol follows our sleep-wake cycle (called the circadian rhythm). Cortisol levels rise at around 6 am and then peak around 8 am. The level rises and falls throughout the entire day and is at its lowest level in the evening, especially when we are asleep. Understanding this pattern gives us an idea when to eat larger meals and when to eat lightly.

4.   Heavier meals should be eaten during the earlier hours of the day, when cortisol levels are higher, to avoid pressuring the adrenal glands. Lighter meals should be eaten during the later parts of the day

when cortisol levels are lower.

5. Throughout the day, schedule healthy meal and snack alternatives. For instance, eating fresh fruits and grains during snack time is better than eating processed food and junk food. These healthier snack alternatives will also help you feel fuller longer and keep you from overeating.

Valuable nutrients for adrenal health

A large part of an Adrenal Reset Power Boost Diet plan involves the use of vitamins, minerals and micronutrients. These can be found in supplements readily purchased from many grocery, health, or drug stores without a prescription. These nutrients are very important for restoring the health of the endocrine system and will promote the health of the adrenal glands.

1. Regulate stress hormones with **vitamins C, E and B complex**. These vitamins will help promote immune system health and help the body cope with stress every day.

2. **Magnesium** is a mineral found in dark-green, leafy vegetables, nuts, seeds, beans, whole grains, yoghurt, bananas and dark chocolate, to name a few. This mineral is

useful for regulating energy to the adrenal glands.

3. **Calcium** is found in cheese, milk, yogurt, seafood, legumes, leafy greens and fruits. Calcium helps in regulating stress and calms the body.

4. Trace minerals such as **zinc, selenium, manganese and iodine** are needed to promote adrenal gland health and reduce stress.

Taking supplements will augment the minimal amounts of nutrients that you get from the food that you take every day. It is impossible to get all the important vitamins and minerals from a daily meal plan. Therefore taking dietary supplements will help.

Important:

If you are suffering from a medical condition or you are currently taking any prescription medication, you should consult your doctor before taking any kind of dietary supplement. Using any kind of over-the-counter supplement has the potential for dangerous interactions and should only be approved or recommended by your physician.

Benefits

The Adrenal Reset Power Boost Diet is a new diet that has been designed from established nutritional data. As the name itself says, this diet will reset your adrenal glands, boost their power, and keep the adrenals healthy and working at their best. It is also a diet that may provide the following benefits:

Improving metabolism

When stress levels rise, the adrenal glands release cortisol and this signals to the body to level up to a heightened state of emergency. The body instinctively tries to protect itself from injury with heightened senses. However, when the body maintains constant levels of stress, the adrenal glands compensate by continuously secreting an increased level of cortisol. Eventually, this can weaken the glands.

Elevated cortisol levels interfere with many metabolic activities in the body including natural functions such as digestion, sleep, immune system functions, and even the production of other kinds of hormones.

All body function is compromised by constant levels of stress.

The Adrenal Reset Power Boost Diet Plan to Improve Metabolism:

1. Allow the adrenal glands to take a break. By consuming fresh, natural and whole foods that are easily digested your glands can rest and recuperate from stress.

2. Allow the adrenal glands to heal. Prolonged exposure to stress wears the adrenal glands down. Following a diet that is composed of healthier food options allows the body to fully benefit from different nutrients such as vitamins and minerals. Taking these nutrients can lead to healthier and well-rested adrenal glands.

3. Allow the adrenal glands to rest with timed food intake. For this kind of diet, food is eaten at specific times during the day, following the natural rise and fall of cortisol levels. There results in less stress for the glands.

Hashimoto's Disease

It is very common for those suffering from Hashimoto's disease to also be afflicted with adrenal fatigue. Hashimoto's disease is a condition in which the immune system attacks the thyroid gland. The thyroid glands are located at the base of the neck just below the larynx. This gland is responsible for producing hormones that are necessary for many of the body's normal activities.

When the thyroid gland becomes inflamed after being attacked, it becomes underactive and leads to a condition called hypothyroidism. The glands produce less hormones because of inflammation and this can result in symptoms such as fatigue, increased sensitivity to cold temperatures, constipation, pale and dry skin, hoarse voice, unexpected weight gain, muscle and joints aches and stiffness, puffy face and excessive menstrual bleeding. People affected by Hashimoto's disease may also suffer from depression and stress.

Adrenal Reset Power Boost Diet for Hashimoto's Disease

Aside from using hormone replacement therapy for Hashimoto's disease, diet plays an important role in regulating thyroid hormones. The Adrenal Reset Power Boost Diet may also help people suffering from Hashimoto's disease. It will:

1. Reduce stress on the thyroid gland. Eating natural, fresh and unprocessed food will ease the work load of the thyroid gland in regulating the body's metabolism. The body will be able to more easily break down food and

convert this into energy for the body to use all day.

2. Allow the thyroid gland to rest and heal. When the thyroid gland is not taxed into producing hormones to help in regulating metabolism, it is able to rest and recuperate.

3. Allow thyroid hormone replacement drugs to work. Hormone replacement treatment (HRT) for Hashimoto's disease works by providing the body with hormones to help in metabolism. Combined with the right diet, HRTs become more effective and may help the thyroid gland to recover more quickly.

4. Provide energy and nutrients that the body needs. The Adrenal Reset Power Boost Diet ensures that the body receives adequate nutrients and energy sources to power the person in daily activities.

Important:

If you are taking medication or hormonal replacement treatment for Hashimoto's disease or other endocrine conditions, consult your doctor before taking any kind of diet or supplement. [But also be aware that many physicians have been slow to acknowledge the problem of

Adrenal Fatigue.]

Sleep disorders

One of the long term effects of adrenal fatigue is poor sleep. When the body is in constant stress, cortisol levels stay high and this can lead to various sleeping disorders such as insomnia and interrupted sleep.

The Adrenal Reset Power Boost Diet Plan to Resolve Sleep Disorders

The ability to get a full, rested night's sleep is important to resetting the adrenal glands. Combining several techniques together should improve your chances of getting the rest that your adrenal glands need.

1. Easing effort on the adrenal glands so cortisol levels gradually return to normal.

2. Allowing the adrenal glands to rest through timed food intake also reduces high levels of cortisol and may help body functions return to normal. Eventually, you will get rid of sleep disorders and normal sleep-wake cycles will return.

3.   By taking in healthy and nutrient-packed food, the body is able to benefit from the vitamins and minerals (such as potassium, magnesium, vitamin D and melatonin) which regulate sleep.

4.   By eating healthy, fresh and whole foods the body is able to generate more energy all day long. Having a constant supply of energy throughout the day helps regulate sleep – wake cycles – this leads to better sleep in the evenings, the best time to relax and sleep for most people.

Important

Some sleep disorders and chronic insomnia may be due to underlying illnesses. If you have been diagnosed with insomnia due to an underlying medical condition, you should consult your doctor before taking any supplement or following any kind of diet plan.

Hypoglycemia

Stress and adrenal fatigue can lead to low blood sugar levels or hypoglycemia. Key hormones that help regulate blood sugar levels – epinephrine, norepinephrine and cortisol – may be affected.

Stress tells the body to be ready for anything and

the body responds by raising blood sugar levels. If, for any reason, the body is unable to meet the demands of stress, hypoglycemia or unhealthy blood sugar swings may occur.

When adrenal hormone levels are low due to the inability of the glands to compensate, it becomes more and more difficult for the body to maintain sugar level balance. The person can become irritable, weak, nervous and sleepless.

The body's natural way of maintaining sugar level balance is a very complex process – any kind of disorder can lead to hypoglycemia and/or adrenal fatigue. Taking medication to resolve this imbalance may not be enough. People who suffer from this condition also need the right kind of diet to boost adrenal function and, eventually, help correct hypoglycemia.

The Adrenal Reset Power Boost Diet Plan for Hypoglycemia

1. Allow the adrenal glands to rest and heal. By eating unprocessed, natural and fresh food, the adrenals do not have to work so hard to produce the hormones that aid in metabolic function. The adrenal glands get the chance to rest and recuperate.

2. Healthy food options or foods that contain nutrients that boost adrenal health can help the glands improve its hormone

secretion leading to improved energy and nutrient absorption.

3. Timing food intake is important for people with hypoglycemia in order to control blood sugar drops and other symptoms of hypoglycemia. Timing is all about eating small frequent meals during the day to take advantage of fluctuating cortisol levels in the body.

4. Eating fresh and natural foods reduces toxin accumulation in the body and this improves adrenal health. Toxins accumulate and may cause all kinds of medical conditions that affect the body's sugar absorption function. Committing to eating fresh and natural meals will reduce this possibility and eventually lead to good adrenal health.

Important:

Hypoglycemia and diabetes can be managed with the use of diet, medication and lifestyle changes. If you have been diagnosed with diabetes, do not take any kind of supplement or use any kind of diet unless it is approved by your doctor. Some cases of hypoglycemia are due to an underlying endocrine condition; stopping the use of medications and using alternative remedies could be dangerous.

Overall improvement to life

There is no doubt that by following the Adrenal Reset Power Boost Diet, you will be able to see and feel an overall improvement in your life. You will feel the changes that you have been longing to happen:

1. You will have more energy during the hours of the day when you most need a boost. You will have more capacity to do all kinds of things now with your new found strength and interest in your surroundings.

2. You will regain your ability to think clearly and make decisions. You won't have to worry about having a foggy mind that could affect your judgment at work and in school.

3. You will be able to bounce back from illness easily, unlike previously when a simple cold could bring you down. Stress and illness are natural life events and therefore you need to be resilient to recuperate unscathed. By following this diet plan, you may be able to completely regain immune system and endocrine health.

4. You enjoy longer periods of being wide

awake and a much more serene sleep at night by following the Adrenal Reset Power Boost Diet plan.

What to eat and what not to eat

You should know by now that the Adrenal Reset Power Boost Diet is about more than just eating the right kinds of food and avoiding the wrong kinds. It is all about eating the best food at the right time and following a good meal plan every day. Here is a list of your best food choices.

Food that you should eat:

Super foods

Not all foods and food groups are created equal. Some foods are known to have higher amounts of nutrients per serving than others and are appropriately called "super foods".

Super foods won't give you super strength, laser vision or the ability to fly, but they will:

1. Boost your immune system health.

2. Improve your digestion and your body's metabolism of foods.

3. Increase your energy levels to

provide what you need every day.

4. Improve your appetite. Super foods are delicious and tasty as well as being very nutritious.

5. Reduce your exposure to toxins with foods are fresh, natural and unprocessed.

The following are some of the best and the tastiest super foods to be included in your everyday diet to boost adrenal health and fight adrenal fatigue:

- Acai juice
- Apples
- Asparagus
- Avocado
- Blackberries
- Broccoli
- Brown rice
- Cauliflower
- Celtic sea salt
- Chicken and turkey
- Coconut
- Fatty fish, such as wild-caught salmon
- Kelp and seaweed
- Kiwi

- Nuts, such as walnuts and almonds
- Olives
- Oysters
- Peanut butter
- Sardines
- Scallops
- Seeds, such as chia and pumpkin
- Soy milk
- Steel-cut oats
- Strawberries
- Sweet potatoes

These are just some of the most popular super foods that you can eat today. Imagine the many meals you can create in a day with the foods on this list – you might even plan your meals in advance for a month. Make sure that you are buying super foods from a well-established retailer or farmer's market so you can be assured of fresh, clean and naturally-grown produce, meats, fish and other types of foods.

High calorie foods

Part of the Adrenal Reset Power Boost Diet is the strategy to eat healthy foods that are high in calories to ensure that you have enough energy throughout the day. High-calorie foods will also contribute to healing and recuperation of your adrenal glands.

The amount of calories that you need daily depends on your age, gender, activity levels and muscle mass. The recommended daily intake is around 2000 calories for most adult individuals.

The following foods are considered to be the healthiest with the most abundant calories:

Food	Calories	Per Cup	Per Table-spoon	Other good sources
Fats and oils Beef tallow, lard, fish oil	902 calories/ 100 g	1849 calories/ 205 g	117 calories/ 13g	Soybean oil, walnut oil, almond oil & coconut oil
Nuts and seeds Macadamia nuts	718 calories/ 100 g	948 calories/ 132 g	201 calories/ 28 g	Pecans, pine nuts, cashew nuts, flaxseeds, chia seeds
Chocolate Dark 70-85% cacao	598 calories/ 100 g	604 calories/ 101 g	167 calories/ 28 g	Dark chocolate 60-69% cacao & dark chocolate 45-59% cacao

Food	Calories	Per Cup	Per Table-spoon	Other good sources
Dried Fruit & fruit juices e.g. Dried prunes / prune juice	339 calories/ 100 g	447 calories / 132 g	224 calories / 66 g	dried cherries, dried blueberries, dried peaches, grape juice, dried apples, pineapple juice and pomegranate juice
Whole grains Whole-wheat pasta, cooked	124 calories/100 g	174 calories / 140 g	87 calories / 70 g	Teff, amaranth, spelt, quinoa, wild rice, soba noodles, bulgur & millet

Food	Calories	Per Cup	Per Table-spoon	Other good sources
Milk, dairy and eggs Goat's cheese, hard	452 calories/ 56 g	254 calories/ 56 g	127 calories/ 28 g	Soft goat's cheese, feta, whole milk, buttermilk, Greek yoghurt, protein powder & whey
Meat Beef brisket, cooked	358 calories/ 100 g	1124 calories/ 314 g	304 calories/ 85 g	Ground pork, turkey bacon, duck meat and skin, veal loin, chicken dark meat & chicken drumsticks

Nutrient-dense foods

There are certain foods that are packed with the nutrient vitamins and minerals that are needed to improve adrenal health:

Vitamin B – rich foods

Foods that are rich in vitamin B complex, especially vitamin B5 (or pantothenic acid) help improve the function of the adrenal glands. A deficiency in pantothenic acid can shrink the adrenal glands and this may cause them to perform poorly, especially during times of stress.

The best sources of pantothenic acid are:

- Animal liver and kidney
- Avocados
- Broccoli
- Chicken
- Egg yolk
- Fish
- Legumes
- Milk
- Mushrooms
- Pork
- Shellfish
- Sweet potatoes
- Yogurt

Vitamin C – rich foods

The body needs vitamin C to boost immunity, improve cardiovascular health and increase adrenal gland health. Vitamin C is needed by the adrenal glands in order to produce the cortisol needed in times of stress.

The following are great sources of vitamin C:

- Berries
- Broccoli
- Brussels sprouts
- Mangoes
- Peaches
- Spring greens
- Tomatoes

L-tyrosine – rich foods

L–tyrosine is needed to reduce the impact of excess stress on the glands. It is important to ease stress on the adrenal glands so that they may heal and become healthier once more.

The following foods are rich in L–tyrosine:

- Avocados
- Bananas
- Chicken
- Dairy products
- Fish
- Legumes
- Nuts
- Oats
- Pork
- Seeds
- Wheat
- Whole grains

Taking nutritional supplements is another way to get these nutrients. People who do not have access to the best and most nutritious foods will be able to improve their dietary intake with the use of supplements. Talk to your doctor for advice on the best supplement brand that is right for you.

Probiotics

Adrenal fatigue can lead to reduced immune system health and therefore it is necessary to find additional ways to help the body fight disease. Using probiotics is one way to keep healthy in spite of adrenal fatigue.

Probiotics are live bacteria as well as yeasts that are known to be good to a person's health. They are essential for digestive system health. Probiotics are considered "good" bacteria as they are able to fight off "bad" or disease-causing bacteria to help keep the digestive system healthy.

Probiotics are essential to the Adrenal Reset Power Boost Diet plan for the following reasons:

1. Losing good bacteria when you take antibiotics is inevitable – probiotics may help replenish your good bacteria population. Antibiotic treatment is often recommended for inflammations and illness; probiotics can help improve overall health during periods of adrenal fatigue.

2. Probiotics prevent illness and infection that could happen when someone is suffering from adrenal fatigue. Avoiding infection is one way to reduce stress on the adrenal glands. Taking a dose of probiotics each day will keep bad bacteria at bay.

3. Adrenal fatigue creates an imbalance in the systems of the body and can make a person feel weak, confused, sleepless, or experience other taxing symptoms. Probiotics can balance good and bad bacteria in the gut and therefore help the body work more efficiently.

There are two types of probiotics, each one has its own benefits. Your doctor will be able to recommend the ideal one that will best suit your condition:

- **Lactobacillus** – this is a common probiotic which is found in yoghurt and in fermented foods. This type of probiotic can help people who are prone to diarrhea or who cannot tolerate lactose in milk.

- **Bifidobacterium** – this is a type of probiotic that is found in some kinds of dairy products and is useful for people with irritable bowel syndrome (IBS).

You may find probiotic drinks, dairy and foods in your local supermarket store. Some probiotics come in easy-to-drink bottles.

The Role of Water

Water cleanses the body inside and out. It is basic to human life and is found in the body's cells and mucous membranes. We are composed ¾ of water, so it makes sense to drink as much as possible each day.

You may also drink natural fruit juices, soups and gelatins, and eat fruits rich in water. Drinking enough water is essential since dehydration can stress the body. Staying hydrated throughout the day improves the adrenals' ability to heal and to recuperate from stress.

Food You Should Avoid

There are some foods that you should avoid while on the Adrenal Reset Power Boost Diet.

Foods that you may be allergic to

As mentioned previously, taxing the adrenal glands further with foods that you are allergic to can worsen your symptoms. Try to avoid these as much as you can.

Sometimes it is very hard to avoid foods that could cause allergies, especially when you are offered an unfamiliar dish or a new type of food. The best rule to remember is to ask questions about the dish:

1. What is the main ingredient? Does it contain any ingredient or food that you are allergic to?

2. If you are certain what type of food you are being offered, yet find yourself still concerned about allergies, refuse the food or simply eat a small amount.

3. Watch out for symptoms after you have taken a few bites.

4. Choose fresh, natural and toxin-free foods. Some people are more sensitive than others. For some even the slightest amounts of chemicals and toxins can lead to allergic reaction. It is always better to be safe than to be sorry.

5. Talk to your doctor about your allergies and how to manage them. The more you are in control of your allergies, the more you will be able to avoid taxing your adrenal glands.

Caffeine

Caffeine can make you feel wide awake and can therefore interfere with your circadian rhythm or your sleep-wake cycle. Caffeine also affects your adrenal glands and can make it hard for them to recover.

If you must drink coffee, take a minimal amount during the mornings. Avoid drinking coffee and black teas, as well as other caffeinated drinks, at least an hour before going to bed.

Sugar and sweeteners

Your body has a tougher time maintaining metabolic functions when you have adrenal fatigue and one of these functions is maintaining sugar levels in the blood. Sweeteners and sugars such as fructose, corn syrup and artificial sweeteners can burden the adrenal glands, causing them to secrete more hormones in order to try to balance sugar levels.

Avoid sweets, sugary foods, cereals, candies and foods that use sugar as additives. The ideal sugar substitute is raw honey; this food will not just sweeten meals, but also provides anti-viral, anti-bacterial, antifungal and antioxidant benefits. Honey also boosts the immune system and can reduce allergic episodes and infections.

Processed, artificially – prepared foods

Almost all processed and artificially-prepared foods are loaded with preservatives and chemicals that will not just tax the adrenals, but may make your symptoms worse. Try to prepare and cook your own foods. Avoid eating out and ordering take out. By shopping, cooking and preparing your own meals, you can significantly reduce the intake of processed foods and – bonus! – improve your cooking skills.

6 PUTTING IT ALL TOGETHER

The most important thing to understand about the Adrenal Reset Power Boost Diet is the importance of putting together everything that you have learned. Remember, that the best way to gain adrenal health is to:

1. Control stress.

2. Follow a sensible diet designed for adrenal fatigue.

3. Use alternative treatments such as exercise and other worthwhile wellness activities.

When you combine all three factors will you be able to protect your adrenal glands from fatigue.

Creating a meal plan

This is a sample meal plan that may inspire you to prepare your own meals for a day or two using the Adrenal Reset Power Boost Diet plan. Note that you can always make any changes or substitutions, as long as the foods that you pick are on the list of foods that you are allowed to eat while on this special diet.

Remember:

1.   Make healthy food choices.

2.   Fresh food is always the best food.

3.   To time food intake.

4.   Choose whole or natural foods.

5.   Pay attention to your allergies.

Breakfast:

- Milk (whole) one glass
- Eggs (boiled or soft-boiled)
- Wheat bread (toasted or as is)
- Tuna in oil or chicken breast
- An apple

Snacks:

- A piece of fruit or a cup of nuts

Lunch:

- Brown rice (one cup)
- Lentil or pea soup
- Salmon with vegetables
- Banana

Snacks:

- A piece of fruit or a cup of nuts

Dinner:

- A broth-based soup
- Brown rice (a cup) or a piece of roll
- Turkey breast
- Mixed vegetable salad
- Watermelon or other fruit in season

Late night snack:

- Cup of frozen berries

Have you noticed anything different about this meal plan? Actually, there is not a huge difference in this meal plan from any healthy diet plan. You will be able to enjoy your meals and you do not have to make food sacrifices.

- You can still enjoy foods that you love to eat

- You do not have to restrain yourself from eating tasty food

- You do not have to purchase expensive food; every food mentioned in this book is readily available from your local store

- Do not worry about finding fresh foods – many grocers and supermarkets already sell these products

And, of course, the most important part of following the Adrenal Reset Power Boost Diet is to enjoy what you are eating! Forget about stress and start enjoying life to the full.

There is no better time to start changing your life than now. Get more energy and achieve more in life with the Adrenal Reset Power Boost Diet plan.

Wake up to a healthier, stress free and good life!

Have you ever felt so weak that you simply cannot get up and go to work? Do you ever get the feeling that you cannot understand the directions given to you or you simply did not understand instructions even though they were only given just a few minutes ago? Have you ever had any unusual cravings? And, did you ever wish that all these weird symptoms would just go away?

Now you can enjoy the life that you once had! The key to a better and more productive life is finally in your hands. Reduce adrenal fatigue now and start living a more stress-free and fulfilling life.

7 CONCLUSION

You have a full life waiting for you! But it will only happen if you take action based on what you have read! Don't waste any more time being tired! Put the information in this book to use so you can take control of your life again, rebalance your hormones and feel energized again.

Use a pencil and blank piece of paper, a notebook, writing program, or even a notation app on your smart phone to create a list of each item in your life that you want to change in order to begin to feel better again:

1. Create an exercise plan that you can stick to. Start slow and work your way up to more vigorous activities.

2. Create a menu for the week and then a shopping list of foods that are going to give you energy and help reduce your symptoms.

3. Make sure you include time in each day to unwind and relax. Many people find joining a yoga class helps. But I am sure you can find plenty of alternatives, even if it is just getting some quiet time to yourself to read a favorite book.

4. Seek out a support group of others who have also experienced Adrenal Fatigue. These are people who know exactly what you have been going through. It is always good to be surrounded by friends who can support you.

5. Stay positive. Look forward to a better tomorrow. If you don't have hope, you will become discouraged. If you can imagine a better tomorrow, you will be encouraged to keep your new-found habits and begin to live a happy life again.

One important fact to reiterate at this stage is that this book has provided you with some general information on the subject of Adrenal Fatigue. It is not intended to and certainly does not replace medical advice from a professional. Always speak to a medical professional before making any major changes to your diet or exercise routine.

Finally, thank you for purchasing this book. If you enjoyed this book, then I'd like to ask you for a favor, would you be kind enough to leave a review for this book at Amazon.com and GoodReads.com? It would be greatly appreciated!

You can follow me at the following social media websites:

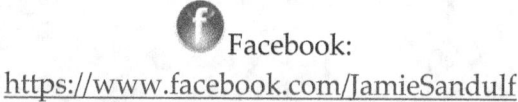
Facebook:
https://www.facebook.com/JamieSandulf

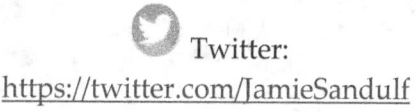
Twitter:
https://twitter.com/JamieSandulf

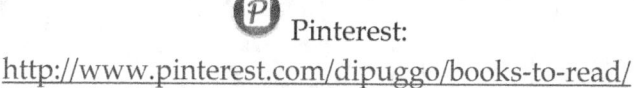
Pinterest:
http://www.pinterest.com/dipuggo/books-to-read/

BONUS BOOK PREVIEW:

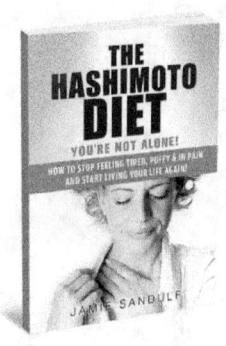

The Hashimoto Diet

**You're Not Alone! How to Stop Feeling
Tired, Puffy & in Pain...and Start
Living Your Life Again!**

Hashimoto's Disease, in which the immune system attacks the thyroid gland, is a lifelong illness. If you have it, it is likely you have suffered from it for quite some time before being able to convince anyone, including doctors, that your symptoms are real and that you have Hashimoto's Disease. It might feel like you are alone in the world and nobody else understands what you are experiencing or how you are suffering. But you are NOT alone! It is estimated that one out of every thousand people, mostly women, are suffering like you (but may be unaware due to misdiagnosis).

Slowly, modern medicine is beginning to recognize this illness and is willing to offer medications to try to treat the symptoms. But medicating the symptoms are not enough. One must also try to eliminate from your systems what is causing the systems if we truly want to recover and begin to live our lives again.

Are you tired of feeling tired all the time? Do you want to stop being depressed? Does the constant joint pain make you feel like doing nothing all day? Annoyed that your face looks puffy and your hair is thinning? Do you want to finally feel warm again and stop freezing even though everyone else is comfortable?

Go to http://amzn.to/1TS1eX9 to read the rest of "*The Hashimoto Diet: You're Not Alone! How to Stop Feeling Tired, Puffy & in Pain...and Start Living Your Life Again!*" at Amazon.com.

ABOUT THE AUTHOR

Jamie Sandulf is a bestselling health book writer of a series of books. Sandulf is passionate about teaching everyone to live healthier lives without being miserable. Sandulf loves to travel for research, but always comes home again to the beloved New England.

Other books by Jamie Sandulf include:

"The Hashimoto Diet: You're Not Alone! How to Stop Feeling Tired, Puffy & in Pain ... and Start Living Your Life Again! "

"Living With An Alcoholic: How To Take Back Control Of Your Relationship and Save The Person You Love"

"Refuse to Live with Prediabetes!: How You Can Lower Your Blood Sugar Levels, Block Insulin Resistance, & Prevent Type II Diabetes Forever!"

"How to Live Longer: Learn the Secrets of Ancient Cultures on How to Live a Longer, Healthier Life"

"Ketogenic Diet: Guide to Quickly Losing Up to 30 Pounds in 30 Days!"

"Carb Cycling: A 28-Day Diet for Women to Boost

Your Metabolism for Accelerated Fat-Burning
Weight Loss"